I0421327

MEDICINAL HERB
ESSENTIALS

The Essential Guide for Growing and Using
Medicinal Herbs for Better Health

Sandi Lane

Limits of Liability, Disclaimer of Warranties & Terms of Use

This book is a general educational information product. As an express condition to reading this book, you understand and agree to following terms. The information and advice contained in this book are not intended as a substitute for consulting with a professional.

The publisher and author make no representations or warranties with respect to the accuracy or completeness of the contents of this work and specifically disclaim all warranties, including without limitation warranties of fitness for a particular purpose. No warranty may be created or extended by sales or promotional materials. The advice and strategies contained herein may not be suitable for every situation. This work is sold with the understanding that the publisher is not engaged in rendering legal, accounting, of the professional services. If professional assistance is required, the services of a competent professional person should be sought. Neither the publisher nor author shall be liable for damages arising therefrom.

ISBN-10: 1514880806
ISBN-13: 978-1514880807

DEDICATION

This book is dedicated to those in search of proven steps and strategies on how to grow some herbs and enjoy their medicinal value.

CONTENTS

INTRODUCTION

People from different parts of the world know what medicinal herbs are because of their long line of uses. Useful in so many ways, many people are in awe of their wonders. For one, they are good for added flavor and serve as taste enhancers for cooking. The medicinal herbs also have aromatic scents that are used in various relaxation and stress relieving techniques. A number of herbs are also perfect for use in the medication of various human ailments and diseases.

The medicinal property of herbs was discovered long ago by the people who inhabited the planet. In fact many incidents are mentioned in biblical stories pertaining to the use of herbs in healing people of their illnesses. Today, along with the advancement of technology, the use of medicinal contents of herbs has evolved as well.

Many types of medicinal herbs are now processed into capsules, syrups, tablets and food supplements. However, many traditional methods are still used by young and old people alike to relieve themselves of pain, sores and other ailments.

This book contains proven steps and strategies on how to grow some herbs and enjoy their medicinal value.
You will be introduced to seven of the most popular herbs that you can easily grow in your garden or even indoors. This book discusses how to grow each one. It also details some of the medical conditions that each herb can treat or cure.

CHAPTER 1 – ALOE VERA

With titles such as Wand of Heaven to Native Americans and Plant of Immortality to the early Egyptians, you just know Aloe Vera is important. Aloe Vera came from Africa and has since been grown all over the world because of the many benefits one can get from it.

For thousands of years Aloe Vera has been lending its hand (or leaves) to people who wish to have beautiful skin and smooth healthy hair. But those are not the only reasons why you should have Aloe Vera planted in your garden.

Medicinal Benefits of Aloe Vera

Aloe Vera is definitely pretty to look at. Its aesthetic value makes it a great addition to any garden. It can also give your home a greener look if you grow them in pots inside. But what makes Aloe Vera an important herb is its medical uses. It has anti-inflammatory, anti-bacterial, and laxative properties.

Ancient people, the Egyptians in particular, knew of the plant's power to make hair beautiful. Until now, shampoos include Aloe Vera as one of their main ingredients. Aloe Vera has the ability to keep hair and scalp healthy. It is useful in treating dandruff and hair loss. Now you don't have to rush to the nearest store when you run out of shampoo. You can simply slice one leaf off your plant and gather the gel inside with a spoon or anything you can scoop it with. Use this gel directly on your hair and scalp before rinsing it off with water.

Cleopatra has been rumored to be a big fan of Aloe Vera. Aside from her hair, she used the gel of the leaves on her skin. It is a good way to moisturize the skin, diminish the appearance of scars, and lighten skin complexion. Aloe Vera can also be used to treat other skin problems such as acne, blisters, eczema, itchiness, and sunburn. Put some of the sap on wounds, insect bites, and burns, as well.

The juice from the leaves can also be used to treat acid reflux, asthma, chronic constipation, Crohn's disease, high cholesterol, inflammation, poor appetite, and digestive problems. Drinking aloe Vera juice is also a popular way of treating ulcerative colitis.

Cultivating Aloe Vera

Planting and growing Aloe Vera is a great way for beginners to learn about gardening. It can be easily grown indoors or outdoors and doesn't need too much of your attention making it a good choice to start your garden with.

With Aloe Vera, you get to experience ACTUALLY growing something in your garden. The fact that it is easy to grow will help enhance your interest in gardening. If you start off with something that is quite difficult to grow, and it turns out unsuccessful, you might lose interest in home gardening altogether. This is one tip that people with no gardening experience should consider. Always start off with herbs that are easy to grow then go on from there as you cultivate your knowledge and experience.

Before loading your garden with Aloe Vera, you have to answer a few questions. First of all, what is the weather condition in your area? Aloe Vera thrives in warm temperature. It grows even better when it gets full sun. If you live in a place that is mostly cold, you may want to grow them in garden pots. This way, you can easily bring them in when the temperature is too cold outside. You can also place wherever in your place there is full sun. You'll know if your plant isn't getting enough sunlight when its leaves are not growing upward. If they turn brown then it's getting too much sun.

What kind of Aloe Vera do you want in your garden? You'd be probably surprised to learn that there are around 500 species of Aloe. You'd want to get your hands on some lace aloe or *Aloe aristata*. This species is one of the best Aloe species to grow indoors. Other variants that you can grow easily are the partridge breast aloe or *Aloe variegata*, and *Aloe barbadensis* which is commonly known as the common aloe.

What about the soil? Aloe Vera likes it soil well-drained. Fill a pot or container with dry and gritty soil and add some fertilizer. You can save up on fertilizer by using the organic kind. It may be a bit more laborious than simply buying chemical fertilizer from the store but going organic is better for the environment. If you have pets, set aside their manure. You can also set aside fruit and vegetable peelings and place them in a compost pit and wait until their good to go. If you want to insist on buying your fertilizer, get the bloom type or the one that says 10-

40-10. Apply this during spring.

How much water does it need? Aloe Vera is made up mostly of water. In fact, it is 95% water! That said, be cautious when you water the plant. Just give it enough. About two cups of water on regular days will be fine. When the temperature is hot and the ground is too dry, make sure to soak the soil completely. Wait until the soil is dry again before watering once more. Observe the plant regularly. If the leaves are not fleshy, it's not getting enough water.

CHAPTER 2 – BASIL

Perhaps one of - if not THE - most popular herb, basil is a must-have in any pantry. Among the different kinds of basil, sweet basil is perhaps the more common. It has flavor that resembles that of anise. Dried basil lends its delightful taste to different dishes while also providing us with nutrients to keep our bodies healthy. Fresh basil tastes even better and is more packed with nutrients. That's why you should be growing it in your garden.

Medicinal Uses of Basil

Basil's main medicinal quality is its anti-inflammatory property. It can be used against arthritis, allergies, bowel inflammation, and other inflammatory conditions. It also has antibacterial properties. The leaves can be used to prevent infections by applying them on the wound. The essential oil extracted from basil is a powerful antioxidant giving the body's immune system an extra boost.

The cinnamanic acid in basil is useful in improving the body's circulation. It has also been discovered to help stabilize sugar making it a natural treatment for diabetes. Basil is also used for treating impotence, infertility, and respiratory problems as well as stress and asthma. It aids in providing relief from colds, fever and flu while also helping against herpes, and heart disease. Research has been positive regarding basil's potential to treat cancer but nothing has been conclusive yet.

It provides the body with lots of vitamins A, K, and C. It is also stacked with calcium, iron, magnesium, and potassium. Aside from being an herbal medicine, basil is also useful in repelling insects. Though basil smells wonderful to us, some insects absolutely abhor it.

Enjoying the benefits of basil is even better if you add the leaves to your cooking. Italian-style pasta dishes work best when topped with basil. You can also make pesto out of basil. Also great for pasta but is even better when you dip your bread in it.

Cultivating Basil

Basil loves the outdoors especially if the condition outside is hot and dry. However, it doesn't do well in the cold. Plant your basil seeds in garden containers that you can easily move. This allows the herb to get full sun during summer and hide indoors during the cold season. Place your plant near the window so it still can get as much sun as possible. If that is still impossible due to the cold, place your herbs in the basement or anywhere as long as they are directly under fluorescent light.

If you prefer to cultivate it in your garden, wait until the frost has gone before starting planting them. You can also grow the seeds indoors first before transplanting them after the frost. Seed germination may take between five to ten days.

This herb requires well-draining soil so the water won't stay too long and cause stress. Water your basil regularly but make sure you don't give it too much. If the leaves at the bottom are starting to turn yellow, ease back on the watering. It is a sign that the plant is under stress most probably due to overwatering. If the leaves are starting to wilt, you need to water a little more.

Basil is an annual herb so you need to take advantage of it while it hasn't lived its life yet. As it grows, prune the leaves to encourage the plant to bush out. Make sure you cut right on top of two opposite leaves. You can also grow more basil plants from cuttings. Just clip off a stem and place the lower end in water. Wait until roots start to grow before planting it on soil. This usually takes two weeks. Harvest time is around ten weeks on the average.

If you don't prune the plant and flowers eventually develop, this means the end is near for your dear herb. Prevent flower from growing or clip off them off so the stem doesn't become woody and stop producing foliage. However, if the herb is near its inevitable death, let the flowers grow and harvest the seeds inside the pods that will eventually develop. These black basil seeds can be planted and grown.

Also, allowing your basil plant to flower leaves you with a wonderful scent coming from these flowers. Basil flowers also attract pollinators so it's basically up to you whether you want to let your herb flower or not.

Sandi Lane

CHAPTER 3 – CHAMOMILE

Chamomile belongs to the *Asteracaea* family of herbs and borrows its name from the Greek words "chamai/kamai" and "melon" which translates to "earth apple". While it does not appear anywhere like an apple, chamomile share its distinct taste and scent. It also shares celebrity status with the fruit. Apple is one of the most popular and tastiest fruits around while chamomile is perhaps the most well-known tea variant in the world.

The two most popular kinds of chamomile are German and Roman. German chamomile, an annual herb that also goes by Blue or Hungarian chamomile, is perhaps the more famous of the two which fans of Roman chamomile will readily argue. German chamomile has a sweet and light taste that makes it a favorite among tea drinkers. Roman chamomile, also known as Noble and Common chamomile, is a perennial herb that is more often used for medicinal purposes rather than for making herbal tea.

Tea made from chamomile is not only regarded for its soothing taste and aroma, it also provides the body with a number of medicinal benefits.

Medicinal Uses of Chamomile

Herbal teas are a staple in Chinese medicine. They have also become a favorite of people who are living a healthy lifestyle. Chamomile has been used as a remedy or cure for a variety of medical conditions for thousands of years. In fact, the early Egyptians were so enamored with the power of chamomile that they offered them to their gods.

Chamomile is not always relegated to teas. The different parts of the herb can be turned into oil which is used in different ways. These extracts can be burned so it may give off a scent that helps relieve stress and allow the mind and body to be at peace. In ancient times and even up to now, chamomile has been used to … the scent of a room.

Chamomile has antibacterial, antibiotic, antispasmodic, antiviral, and antiseptic properties. It can also be used as a disinfectant. This herb has been used throughout history as a cure for stomach problems such as heartburn, flatulence, and indigestion. You can also take it to treat cough, fever, bronchitis, diarrhea, skin lesions, herpes, skin inflammations, and issues with the liver and gallbladder. Some studies have shown that chamomile may also help lower blood sugar which is necessary for people suffering from diabetes. A cup of chamomile tea taken before bed is also said to help out against nightmares. This is probably because of its soothing effect that calms the mind before you fall asleep.

Cultivation of Chamomile

If you're planning on cultivating chamomile at home, you better start off with either the Roman chamomile (*Chamaemelum nobile*) or the German chamomile (*Matricaria recutita*). These two species of the herb are the most common.

Chamomile is grown from the seeds. They like full sun but may suffer if the temperature gets too high. Plant them somewhere that it can get full sun but can still get some shade later in the day.

Scatter the seeds over sandy soil that is slightly acidic. The soil should also be well-draining. To give your seeds a better chance of growth, apply some fertilizer or better yet, compost. There is no need to cover the scattered seeds with soil. There is a need, however, to start planting after frost. You'll be leaving the seeds exposed and you don't want them getting buried under snow, right?

Allow the seeds to germinate for two weeks. Once they become seedlings, thin them. This will allow the chamomile seedlings with the best chance of surviving to thrive. Water them regularly even if they are drought-resistant. Doing so will allow the seedlings to stay upright and for the stems to become sturdy.

Wait until the flowers are fully opened before harvesting them. You can make tea out of these freshly picked flowers. Another option is to dry them. You must take off the stems and leaves before drying the flowers.

Sandi Lane

CHAPTER 4- OREGANO

From the mint or *Lamiaceae* family comes the genus *Origanum*, more popular as oregano. This perennial herb's name is derived from the Greek words "oros" meaning "mountain" and "ganos" which is "joy". It also goes by as wild marjoram in some parts of the world.

Oregano is a familiar face in kitchens. It lends its spicy and sometimes sweet flavors to different dishes. The herb has different subspecies that is why pinpointing a specific taste is quite difficult. Every kind of oregano has a different taste and aroma.

Medicinal Uses of Oregano

Oregano oil extract may be used for a variety of ailments. It is a potent anti-bacterial because of the *carvacrol* and *thymol* it contains. It can be handy in fighting off bacterial infections caused by *Staphylococcus aureus* and *Pseudomonas aeruginosa*. Aside from the phytonutrients mentioned, oregano also contains *rosmarinic acid*, which along with *thymol*, makes it a powerful anti-oxidant, as well.

Oregano is likewise used against digestive and respiratory problems. Furthermore, it can treat fungal infections and other infections caused by parasites. Oregano oil may also be applied topically on the skin to provide relief for muscle and joint pain while also effective against psoriasis and dandruff. If you're out of citronella oil, you can also use oregano oil to keep insects at bay.

This herb can also help your body ward off free radicals thanks to being a potent antioxidant. It has also been proven in a lab that oregano can kill *Listeria monocytogenes* and MRSA. Another study, this time conducted in Germany, found out that oregano can also be a potential cancer cure. The beta-caryophyllin in oregano may also work against medical disorders such as osteoporosis.

You can get your daily nutrient fix from this herb. Oregano is high in Vitamin K which is vital in bone growth and blood clotting proteins. It also provides you with Vitamin E, calcium, iron, manganese, fiber, and omega fatty acids.

Oregano may be used to treat headaches, fatigue, toothache, acne, dandruff, and allergies. It has been tries against heart problems, intestinal parasites, and lesser things such as dandruff and allergic.

Cultivating Oregano

Get your hands on some oregano seeds. Start sowing them indoors in containers. It will take seven to fourteen days for the oregano seeds to germinate. Once they do, you can transplant the seedlings to your garden.

Oregano prefers an area that gets full sun. If your place has a hotter than usual climate, you may want to place your herbs somewhere it can get shade during the afternoon. Too much sun may be detrimental to their growth. The same can be said about the cold. Cover your herbs with mulch to prevent them from freezing.

In eleven to thirteen weeks, you can harvest your oregano leaves and even the flowers and enjoy them on various dishes particularly on Greek cuisine. You can use them fresh or dry them before using.

Sandi Lane

CHAPTER 5 – TURMERIC

Indian cuisine would not be the same if not for this herb. Turmeric is responsible for the yellow hue of most of the dishes that was popularized by India. Turmeric looks like ginger but has a brighter yellow color. It is known for its pungent taste and distinct smell. While a popular ingredient in Indian and Asian cooking, turmeric was used in ancient times as a natural dye. Buddhist monks of yore gave their robes that distinctive color using dye made out of turmeric. Indian wedding then wouldn't be complete without the bride and groom being colored using a paste made from the herb.

Medicinal Uses of Turmeric

Turmeric is a staple in Ayurvedic medicine and has been used to treat a variety of ailment for thousands of years. It was effective then in treating wounds and is still useful today because of its antibacterial property. It is also an antiseptic which makes it even more useful for treating wounds, burns, and cuts.

For those who wish to lose a few pounds, turmeric may be of help. This herb contains cucurmin, its active ingredient. Cucurmin can help in promoting digestion which leads to better metabolism of fat. Once consumed, cucurmin acts by stimulating the gallbladder which is the key to weight loss. It also helps control the cholesterol level in our body.

Turmeric is also great for the skin and we're not just talking about coloring the skin as people back in the day did when they got hitched. This herb can be applied topically on the skin to treat acne and psoriasis. It might as well be a new mom's best friend as it is effective and making those stretch marks disappear or lighten at the very least. It may also be used to exfoliate the skin and lessen the visibility of wrinkles. Add powdered turmeric into your favorite moisturizer or other skin products or make a face pack with it to easily reap the benefits of this magnificent herb.

A number of studies have been conducted to try to determine if turmeric has a positive effect on medical conditions such as Alzheimer's disease and cancer. In the case of cancer, one research used mice as the subjects. These rodents were made sick with breast cancer and then treated using turmeric. Results showed a positive effect against the disease. Another test involved prostate cancer. Here, it was discovered that a combination of turmeric and cauliflower was effective in inhibiting the growth of the cancer.

Tests determining the effect of the herb on Alzheimer's disease were also successful to some extent. Turmeric prevented amyloid plaque buildup in the brain of the subjects. This action, in turn, hinders the progression of Alzheimer's disease. While nothing is conclusive as of yet, the results gathered have been positive and the potential is quite exciting. A few more studies and we might be seeing an effective cure against this disease.

Turmeric also has potent anti-inflammatory properties. It has been found to be helpful in treating arthritis and providing relief from its symptoms. Turmeric may also be used for detoxification, and consequently, in helping out the liver.

This herb has also been known to aid in treating depression and lessening the physical effects of a stress. Turmeric likewise prevents metastases.

There are a number of ways you can use turmeric for its medicinal qualities. As mentioned, it can be made into a face pack or mixed with moisturizers to keep your skin healthy and looking young. You can also make tea out of it. Powdered or ground turmeric is available in the market and can be made into tea. But if you wish to have a fresh cup every day, you can simply place a chunk of turmeric in a cup of hot water and let it steep. Alternatively, you can grind the turmeric before adding it into the water. If turmeric tea is not your cup of... tea, you can always make juice out of this herb. Because turmeric has a strong taste, you may need to mix it with tastier ingredients – say lemon and honey – for it to be more palatable.

Cultivating Turmeric

Unlike the rest of the herbs in this list, turmeric cannot be grown from seeds. It is cultivated from its rhizomes or roots. To get your turmeric garden going, look for turmeric roots that are fresh, plump, and has lots of buds. They are usually available at your local market. You can also try the local nursery.

Once you've chosen your turmeric roots, there's two ways you can go about planting them. First, you can plant the whole thing. Just make sure you place the side that has the most buds upwards. The other method is to cut off the buds and plant them one by one.

Turmeric thrives in well-draining soil. Prepare your soil first by moistening it a bit so tilling will be a bit easier. You can likewise use garden pots or containers filled with soil. Dig two inch deep holes that are at least a foot apart. Afterwards, place a root in each hole with the buds facing upwards. If you're using pots, place them in an area that gets full sun. Turmeric likes the temperature to be somewhere between 20 to 30°C. You can transplant the sprouts later on to your garden if you wish.

Water them regularly but be careful not to overwater. Root rot is one of the major problems in growing turmeric and too much water will do just that. You'll notice sprouts after a few weeks but it will take around eight to ten months before you can start harvesting the roots.

CHAPTER 6 – THYME

Thyme is of the essence if you talk about Mediterranean cuisine. Originally from Southern Europe, thyme has gone a long way to become one of the most common herbs found in every kitchen around the globe. In France, this herb is an important ingredient for their *bouquet garni* which is a mixture of different herbs. The Arabs, have their own version called *za'atar*. This combination of herb and spice mixture with lots of thyme and oregano goes well with flatbread. For the rest of the world, thyme is often used on soups and stews while also lending its distinct taste to many a vegetable dish.

There are different varieties of thyme. The common thyme is what most are familiar with though lemon thyme and wild thyme are also quite well-known.

In ancient times, Greeks burned thyme like an incense to provide a wonderful aroma in their temples. Egyptians, meanwhile, used thyme for embalming their pharaohs. While thyme is not used for embalming anymore, it retains its importance especially in cooking. But what is often overlooked is that thyme possesses medicinal qualities that benefit everyone.

Medicinal Value of Thyme

For the longest time, thyme has been used as a cure for various ailments. It was mainly used in ancient times for treating different respiratory problems. It can be made into tea to provide relief to cough and chest congestion. As time went by, people realized that thyme can be useful against other medical issues concerning the respiratory system such as asthma, laryngitis, sinus infection, and even bronchitis.

What makes this herb effective against respiratory issues is the naturally occurring compound terpenoid. This natural chemical in thyme enables the herb to relax the bronchi and enhance the function of the cilia while also acting as an expectorant. Terpenoids also allow thyme to fight off or at least deter cancer, as some study shows.

The secret to thyme's medicinal value, aside from the terpenoids, is its active ingredients. Its main active ingredient is *thymol* which mostly accounts for its healing powers. Its other components – *borneol, carvacolo, and geraniol* – contribute, as well.

Thymol is also an ingredient of most mouthwashes. If you're suffering from halitosis or simply want to prevent having bad breath, consuming thyme may help a lot. Thyme is a potent antibacterial which makes it capable of getting rid of germs and bacteria that causes one's mouth to smell. It is also useful against other bacterial infection including acne. Because thyme has antiseptic and antifungal properties, as well, it may be used to treat different skin conditions.

Thyme is also currently being considered as a potential cure for cancer. Studies done have proven that the herb aids in preventing the Big C. Scientists discovered that the rosmarinic and ursolic acids in the herb can fight off the disease.

Cultivating Thyme

Thyme, like basil, is rather easy to cultivate. It can grow in a hot environment, on mountain highlands, and even in places that experience frost.

If you want to grow thyme from seeds, you can do so. But if you want to skip having to wait for it them to germinate, you can purchase seedlings from nurseries and greenhouses.

Like most herbs, thyme thrives under full sun. Find a place in your garden where the sun shines especially in the morning and gets a bit of shade in the afternoon. This way, your plant won't suffer during times that the temperature is extremely hot. Better yet, grow them in plants so you can easily handle them and place them where they need to be. If frost looms, simply place lots of mulch on the soil to protect their roots from freezing.

The soil should be sandy and well-draining. Thyme can survive even if you don't water them at a regular rate. Water them frequently only when the condition is extremely hot and dry. Otherwise, just water them every two days.

Sandi Lane

CHAPTER 7 – PEPPERMINT

Herbs are known for their smell and probably the best-smelling of the lot is peppermint. Who doesn't love smelling its menthol scent? It's so soothing that you'd think you're in Antarctica or something.

Peppermint is a perennial herb which is a cross between spearmint and watermint. It originated from Middle East and Europe but is now cultivated worldwide.

Medicinal Uses of Peppermint

Peppermint is another one of the herbs used in medicine during the early times. If you haven't figured it out yet, ancient healers depended on nature for their craft. These early doctors may be scratching their heads or turning in their graves just thinking about all the medicines manufactured by giant pharmaceuticals that people use nowadays. Back in those days, people simply drank herbal teas, pounded plant parts to make paste, or directly scrubbed herbs on themselves to treat an ailment.

Peppermint is one of those herbs that something as simple as their scent can help cure an illness – physical or otherwise. The relaxing aroma of the herb helps sooth headaches. It may also provide relief for toothache. Using peppermint oil on the body will lessen the degree of hurt you'd normally feel because of muscle and nerve pain.

This herb is probably more known as a cure for coughs and cold. Cough medicines today usually include peppermint as one of its ingredients. However, you don't need to rely on such medicines. Simply drop some peppermint leaves in boiling water and let it steep for a while. The result should be a tasty and healthy cup of tea. If you are suffering from a congested nose, you can inhale the scent of peppermint oil or place leaves in a bowl of extremely hot water. Cover your head, which is right above the tub of hot water, with a blanket and inhale the steam. The steam with the help of peppermint will help you breathe easier.

Indigestion, dyspepsia, and other problems with the digestive tract can be treated with peppermint. Flatulence, irritable bowel syndrome, and stomach pain will gradually go away if you employ the services of dear peppermint. It also lends a hand (or a leaf) against morning sickness, inflammations in the mouth and throat, diarrhea, rashes, and liver problems.

Cultivating Peppermint

Peppermint can grow basically anywhere. It also doesn't matter what the weather condition is. It grows even in wet conditions. In fact, peppermint grows better in moist areas. But if you really wish to be successful in growing peppermint, you should know what the right conditions are.

First of all, you need an area that has moderately rich soil. It is also better if there is partial shade so the herb will stay safe during overly hot temperatures. Prepare the soil by tilling it. Then gather some boards and bury them at least six inches down. The boards should be standing and should create a box under the ground. The purpose of this is to prevent peppermint from invading other areas in your garden. This herb likes to take over the place. If left unchecked, peppermint may spread all over your garden and these walls made from the board will help prevent it from happening.

Once the soil is ready, you can proceed to planting the seeds. A better alternative is to plant peppermint cuttings as they will grow faster. Bury the bottom part of each cutting at least two inches deep and half a foot apart. This will give each plant ample space to grow.

Water the herbs regularly by giving them around six inches worth of water weekly. Remember to clip off the buds as the plant grows. By cutting of the budding tips, the growth of the peppermint will spread and become bushy. Once the herb reaches at least ten inches high, harvesting the leaves can commence. If you insist on harvesting beforehand, the plant may weaken and eventually die.

Please Leave a Review

Finally, if you enjoyed this book, please take the time to share your thoughts and post a review on Amazon. It would be greatly appreciated.

That review and feedback will help me improve the content in my books – and make each and every one more relevant and helpful to you.

Thank you again and good luck!

Sandi Lane